MW00884207

No Flour No Sugar Cookbook Vol. 2

More Quick and Easy Clean Eating Recipes for Weight Loss and a Healthier You

Madison Miller

Copyrights

All rights reserved © Madison Miller and The Cookbook Publisher. No part of this publication or the information in it may be quoted from or reproduced in any form by means such as printing, scanning, photocopying, or otherwise without prior written permission of the copyright holder.

Disclaimer and Terms of Use

Effort has been made to ensure that the information in this book is accurate and complete. However, the author and the publisher do not warrant the accuracy of the information, text, and graphics contained within the book due to the rapidly changing nature of science, research, known and unknown facts, and internet. The author and the publisher do not hold any responsibility for errors, omissions, or contrary interpretation of the subject matter herein. This book is presented solely for motivational and informational purposes only.

The recipes provided in this book are for informational purposes only and are not intended to provide dietary advice. A medical practitioner should be consulted before making any changes in diet. Additionally, recipe cooking times may require adjustment depending on age and quality of appliances. Readers are strongly urged to take all precautions to ensure ingredients are fully cooked in order to avoid the dangers of foodborne illnesses. The recipes and suggestions provided in this book are solely the opinion of the author. The author and publisher do not take any responsibility for any consequences that may result due to following the instructions provided in this book.

ISBN: 978-1973792178

Printed in the United States

Avant-Propos

You have a plan, and that plan is to finally heal your body, lose the excess weight that you've been carrying around, and enjoy a burst of energy that you haven't had in years. There are plenty of diets that claim to help you achieve this. The problem is that most of those diets don't address the real problem. The real problem with our diets today can be summed up with two words: 'sugar' and 'flour.' These two ingredients alone contribute to many of the chronic diseases we suffer from. The No Sugar, No Flour dietary plan helps you to regain your health and recharge your energy naturally. This plan is different from your standard low carb plans and *there are no complicated calculations*. All you need is the desire and willpower to cut out two simple ingredients, along with the inspiration for some creative, delicious meals that won't leave you feeling like you are missing a single thing.

That is where this book comes in. Inside these pages, you will find recipes for every meal, using ingredients that fuel and heal your body, rather than depleting it. These recipes will help cure your ailments, help you lose weight, and help you to once again feel healthy and youthful. All the flavor – and none of the bad flour and sugar – is what you will find in these recipes. This book is a delicious adventure in health, vitality, and unbelievable flavor.

Contents

Introduction

What do you notice as you walk through your local grocery store? Are the aisles brimming with fresh produce and meats? Unfortunately, these sections of most grocery stores account for only a small portion of the space, compared with the aisles filled with processed, pre-made foods. Many pre-packed foods claim to be healthy options, and in fact, some of them are. However, the truth remains that today our diets are those of convenience, where we often must choose between foods that are fresh, or foods that are quick to prepare, foods that are nutritious, or those that will allow us to feed our families on a budget. Here we have the central point of all our nutritious and dietary woes – our diets are filled with processed foods, many in the form of simple carbohydrates.

Carbohydrates are a necessity. Your body depends upon them to create energy and provide the fuel that will get you through your day. There are two types of carbohydrates: simple and complex. As we are coming off what seems to be the tail end of the low carbohydrate diet craze, we have learned that while carbohydrates are necessary, they are not all created equal. Rather than shunning all carbohydrates, we have learned that it is necessary to discriminate among them. Rather than living off bacon and cheddar cheese, we have learned that a well-rounded diet, rich in complex carbohydrates, allows us to not only lose weight, but also regulate our blood sugar, lower blood pressure, and calm down the over-reactive inflammatory response that years of processed foods has caused. We have learned from our mistakes and we are in the process of building a new, healthier dietary philosophy in the process.

This is where no flour, no sugar eating comes into the picture. Simple carbohydrates come from foods containing processed flour and white sugar. These two ingredients alone are thought to be responsible for a myriad of diseases, including

- Chronic Fatigue
- Diabetes
- High Cholesterol
- Cardiac Disease
- Obesity
- Depression
- Anxiety
- Skin Disorders
- Autoimmune Diseases
- Dementia
- Cancer

In addition to this, foods that contain flour and sugar are more likely to be nutritionally void. One study showed that if you were to live off only white bread for two months, you would suffer from such severe malnutrition that your organs could begin to shut down. During the process of producing and refining white flour, nearly one hundred vitamins and minerals are removed from the wheat kernel. Now, stop and think about how many foods we eat, without even thinking about it, that contain flour or sugar among their main ingredients? It is no wonder that as a society we suffer from so many serious, chronic health conditions. The solution to this problem is a simple one: you simply eliminate flour and sugar from your diet.

While the idea of cutting out flour and sugar completely might sound daunting, the truth is that it really isn't that difficult. It's all about reprogramming your mind and your taste buds to favor natural flavors rather than synthetic ones. It's about learning to appreciate the luscious sweetness of fresh fruit over the overly sweet, sticky chocolate cake. It's about learning to choose whole grains such as millet or quinoa over a plateful of pasta. These are small adjustments that, over time, will make incredibly positive changes in your health.

This book has been designed to help you learn and experience just how delicious no flour, no sugar meals can be. There are two things that each of these recipes have in common. The first is that they contain no refined white sugar or flour. The second is that they are each a delicious example of healthy, natural, and wholesome cooking. This book is divided by type of meal, presenting you with tasty options for every meal from breakfast to a little sweet treat at the end of the day. From this point forward, every meal and every snack will be an experience, a natural, wholesome flavor sensation that will leave your body and your soul satisfied. Enjoy.

Note: Some people will choose to follow this eating plan simply because they want to eat healthier, while others will follow it because their immediate health depends on it. Some recipes include OPTIONAL ingredients such as honey or white wine that will be reduced during cooking. Note the word 'optional.' A little natural honey is much better than refined white sugar, but it can be left out altogether if you are avoiding all types of sugar for health reasons. The recipes that contain these optional ingredients are just as delicious without them as they are with them, so first and foremost always follow your own dietary guidelines and adjust these recipes to suit yourself as needed.

Breakfast Dishes

Pear, Spinach, and Goat Cheese Omelet

Servings: 2
Prep Time: 10 minutes
Cook Time: 10 minutes

Ingredients
1 tablespoon butter or margarine, divided

1 cup pear, thinly sliced

3 cups spinach, chopped

½ teaspoon nutmeg

½ teaspoon salt

1 teaspoon coarse ground black pepper

4 eggs, beaten

½ cup goat cheese

Directions
1. Heat half the butter in a medium-sized skillet or omelet pan over medium heat.
2. Add the pear and cook, stirring frequently, for 1 minute.
3. Next, add the spinach and season the mixture with the nutmeg, salt, and black pepper. Continue cooking until the spinach is wilted and the pears are tender.
4. Using a slotted spoon, remove the contents from the skillet and set them aside.
5. Add the remaining butter to the skillet and increase the heat to medium high.

6. Pour the eggs into the skillet. (Note: You can add all the eggs at once and divide up the finished dish into two portions, or you can add half the eggs, cook, add the fillings and the repeat for the second omelet.)
7. Swirl the skillet to ensure that the eggs cover the bottom surface.
8. As the edges of the eggs begin to set, carefully lift up the edges to allow more liquid egg to flow to the outside.
9. Repeat this one or two more times, until the egg is mostly set.
10. Spread the pear and spinach mixture out over half of the omelet.
11. Sprinkle goat cheese over the spinach.
12. Cook for 1-2 minutes, or until the cheese begins to melt.
13. Carefully fold the other side of the omelet over onto the side with the filling.
14. Remove the omelet from the skillet and serve immediately.

Nutritional Information (per serving)

Calories 321.6, Total Fat 21.6 g, Saturated Fat 11.0 g,
Total Carbs 13.2 g, Dietary Fiber 3.2 g, Sugars 7.7 g, Protein 19.4 g

Sweet Potato Apricot Breakfast Muffins

Servings: 18
Prep Time: 10 minutes
Cook Time: 30 minutes

Ingredients
1 ½ cups sweet potato, mashed

4 eggs

1 ½ cups raw almonds

2 teaspoons baking powder

2 teaspoons cinnamon

1 teaspoon ground ginger

½ teaspoon coriander

1 cup zucchini, shredded

1 cup apple, shredded

1 cup unsweetened shredded coconut

1 cup dried apricots, chopped

½ cup dates, chopped

1 cup walnuts, chopped

Directions
1. Preheat the oven to 375°F and line or oil and flour 18 standard-sized muffin cups.
2. Place almonds in a food processor and grind finely.
3. In a bowl, combine the sweet potatoes with the eggs, almond flour, baking powder, cinnamon, ginger, and coriander. Mix just until blended.
4. Next, fold in the zucchini, apple, coconut, apricots, dates, and walnuts.

7

5. Spoon the batter into the prepared muffin cups.
6. Place the muffins in the oven and bake for 30-35 minutes, or until set in the center.
7. Remove from the oven and let cool slightly before serving.

Nutritional Information (per serving)

Calories 178.8, Total Fat 11.7 g, Saturated Fat 3.1 g,
Total Carbs 16.6 g, Dietary Fiber 3.6 g, Sugars 10.0 g, Protein 5.1 g

Savory Mushroom Breakfast Muffins

Servings: 10
Prep Time: 10 minutes
Cook Time: 20 minutes

Ingredients

1 cup mushrooms, chopped

2 cloves garlic, crushed and minced

2 ½ cups almond flour

1 teaspoon baking soda

1 tablespoon fresh thyme, chopped

1 teaspoon sea salt

1 teaspoon coarse ground black pepper

3 eggs

⅓ cup cooked sweet potato, mashed

2 tablespoons olive oil

½ cup walnuts, chopped

½ cup brie, cubed

Directions

1. Preheat the oven to 350°F and line or oil and flour 10 standard-sized muffin cups.
2. Spray a skillet with cooking oil and place it over medium heat.
3. Add the mushrooms and garlic to the skillet and sauté for 2-3 minutes, or until the mushrooms are tender. Remove the skillet from the heat and set it aside.
4. In a bowl, combine the almond flour, baking soda, thyme, sea salt, and black pepper. Mix well.

5. In a separate bowl, combine the eggs, sweet potato, and olive oil. Mix well.
6. Add the dry ingredients to the wet ingredients and blend until just combined.
7. Fold in the mushrooms, walnuts, and brie.
8. Spoon the batter into the prepared muffin cups.
9. Bake for approximately 20 minutes, or until the set in the center.
10. Let cool slightly before serving.

Nutritional Information (per serving)
Calories 252.8, Total Fat 22.0 g, Saturated Fat 3.4 g,
Total Carbs 7.7 g, Dietary Fiber 3.6 g, Sugars 1.8 g, Protein 9.7 g

Griddle Cakes with Mascarpone Blueberry Topping

Servings: 4
Prep Time: 10 minutes
Cook Time: 15 minutes

Ingredients
4 eggs

⅔ cup unsweetened applesauce

½ cup almond flour

1 teaspoon baking powder

½ teaspoon ground cinnamon

½ teaspoon ground ginger

½ teaspoon pure vanilla extract

1 tablespoon honey (optional)

½ cup mascarpone cheese

1 teaspoon orange zest

½ cup orange juice, divided

1 cup blueberries

Directions
1. In a bowl, combine the eggs and the applesauce. Mix until blended.
2. In a separate bowl, combine the almond flour, baking powder, cinnamon, and ginger. Mix well.
3. Add the dry ingredients to the wet ingredients, along with the vanilla extract and the honey, if you are using it. Mix until blended and set aside.

4. In a small bowl, combine the mascarpone cheese, orange zest, and about two teaspoons of the orange juice. Mix well and set aside.
5. In a small saucepan, combine the blueberries and the remaining orange juice. Heat over medium to medium high, stirring frequently, until the blueberries begin to soften and break down. Reduce the heat to low and simmer while you are cooking the griddle cakes.
6. Prepare a griddle with a light coating of cooking spray and heat it over medium-low heat.
7. Once the griddle is warmed, spoon approximately ¼ cup of the batter onto the griddle for each cake.
8. Cook for approximately 3 minutes before flipping and cooking for an additional 2-3 minutes, or until golden brown and set in the center.
9. Serve the griddle cakes with the mascarpone cheese and warm blueberry topping.

Nutritional Information (per serving)
Calories 281.1, Total Fat 19.8 g, Saturated Fat 5.8 g,
Total Carbs 15.7 g, Dietary Fiber 2.9 g, Sugars 10.9 g, Protein 9.4 g

Deviled Egg Scramble

Servings: 2
Prep Time: 10 minutes
Cook Time: 10 minutes

Ingredients
1 tablespoon butter or margarine

½ cup sweet yellow onion, diced

½ cup roasted red peppers, chopped

1 tablespoon capers

5 eggs, beaten

1 tablespoon Dijon mustard

1 tablespoon prepared horseradish

1 teaspoon fresh chives, chopped

Directions
1. Heat the butter or margarine in a skillet over medium heat. Once melted, add the sweet yellow onion and sauté for 2 minutes.
2. Add the roasted red peppers and the capers. Cook, stirring frequently, for an additional 2-3 minutes, or until the onions are softened and beginning to caramelize.
3. To the beaten eggs, add the Dijon mustard and the prepared horseradish. Whisk together until well blended.
4. Spread the onion and pepper mixture out over the surface of the skillet.
5. Pour the egg mixture into the skillet.
6. Continue cooking, scrambling the eggs until they are cooked to your desired doneness.
7. Transfer the eggs to serving plates and garnish with chives before serving.

Nutritional Information (per serving)
Calories 270.8, Total Fat 17.9 g, Saturated Fat 7.7 g,
Total Carbs 8.0 g, Dietary Fiber 1.6 g, Sugars 2.6 g, Protein 17.0 g

Portabella Breakfast Sandwich

Servings: 2
Prep Time: 5 minutes
Cook Time: 10 minutes

Ingredients
4 large portabella mushroom caps

1 tablespoon olive oil

½ teaspoon sea salt

½ teaspoon coarse ground black pepper

2 eggs, prepared to liking

¼ cup goat cheese

½ cup roasted red pepper, sliced

2 cups arugula

½ avocado, sliced

Directions
1. Liberally brush both sides of the mushroom caps with the olive oil and season them with the sea salt and coarse ground black pepper.
2. Place the mushroom caps in a skillet over medium heat.
3. Cook for 2-3 minutes per side, or until tender, but still firm.
4. Remove the mushroom caps from the skillet and immediately spread them with the goat cheese.
5. Take two of the mushroom caps and stack the eggs, roasted red pepper slices, arugula, and avocado on top.
6. Top each stack with a remaining mushroom cap.
7. Serve immediately.

Nutritional Information (per serving)
Calories 409.9, Total Fat 31.2 g, Saturated Fat 8.6 g,
Total Carbs 19.4 g, Dietary Fiber 12.7 g, Sugars 4.6 g, Protein 20.3 g

Orange Creamsicle Breakfast Porridge

Servings: 2
Prep Time: 5 minutes
Cook Time: 10 minutes

Ingredients
1 cup unsweetened coconut milk

½ cup unsweetened shredded coconut

1 vanilla bean, scraped, insides only

½ cup orange juice

1 teaspoon orange zest

¼ cup almond flour

2 tablespoons flax meal

2 tablespoons chia seeds

1 tablespoon honey (optional)

Fresh fruit for serving (optional)

Directions
1. Combine all the ingredients in a large saucepan over medium heat, including the honey if you choose to include it.
2. Cook, stirring frequently, for 10-12 minutes, or until the porridge reaches your desired thickness.
3. Serve with fresh, chopped fruit, if desired.

Nutritional Information (per serving)
Calories 331.5, Total Fat 25.9 g, Saturated Fat 8.2 g,
Total Carbs 21.4 g, Dietary Fiber 11.6 g, Sugars 6.9 g, Protein 10.5 g

Lunch and Brunch Recipes

Blue Buffalo Chicken Wraps

Servings: 4
Prep Time: 10 minutes
Cook Time: 10 minutes

Ingredients
¼ cup mayonnaise

¼ cup buttermilk

2 cloves garlic, crushed and minced

2 teaspoons fresh chives, chopped

½ cup blue cheese crumbles

1 pound boneless, skinless chicken breast, cubed

½ teaspoon salt

1 teaspoon coarse ground black pepper

1 teaspoon granulated garlic

1 tablespoon butter

1 cup celery, diced

½ cup cayenne pepper sauce

1 avocado, sliced

4-8 large butter lettuce leaves

Directions

1. In a bowl, combine the mayonnaise, buttermilk, garlic, and chives. Using a whisk, blend together until well mixed. Add the blue cheese crumbles and stir. Set aside.
2. Season the chicken with the salt, black pepper, and granulated garlic.
3. Heat the butter in a large skillet over medium heat.
4. Add the chicken and cook for 1-2 minutes.
5. Next, add the celery and stir. Cook, stirring frequently, for 5-7 minutes, or until the chicken is browned and cooked through.
6. Pour the cayenne pepper sauce into the skillet and stir, making sure the chicken is evenly coated in the sauce.
7. Lay out the butter lettuce leaves. You can use one per wrap, or use two for a slightly larger, more secure wrap.
8. Spoon a serving of chicken into the center of each leaf.
9. Top each portion with the blue cheese dressing and avocado slices.
10. Wrap and serve immediately.

Nutritional Information (per serving)

Calories 375.5, Total Fat 25.1 g, Saturated Fat 7.9 g,
Total Carbs 6.5 g, Dietary Fiber 3.7 g, Sugars 1.2 g, Protein 31.2 g

Caprese Muffins

Servings: 6
Prep Time: 15 minutes
Cook Time: 30 minutes

Ingredients
½ cup sundried tomatoes, chopped

2 cloves garlic, crushed and minced

1 cup fresh basil, chopped

1 cup zucchini, shredded with excess moisture removed

½ cup almond flour

1 tablespoon flax seed meal

1 teaspoon sea salt

1 teaspoon coarse ground black pepper

¼ teaspoon baking powder

2 eggs, lightly beaten

½ cup fresh mozzarella, shredded

Directions
1. Preheat the oven to 350°F and line or grease and flour six standard-sized muffin cups.
2. In a blender or food processor, combine the sundried tomatoes, garlic, and basil. Pulse until a paste forms.
3. Place the zucchini in a bowl and add the mixture from the blender. Mix well.
4. In a separate bowl, combine the almond flour, flax seed meal, sea salt, coarse ground black pepper and baking powder.
5. Add the dry ingredients and the eggs to the vegetable mixture. Mix well.

19

6. Stir in the fresh mozzarella cheese.
7. Spoon the batter evenly into the prepared muffin cups.
8. Place the muffins in the oven and bake for 30-35 minutes, or until set in the center.
9. Let cool before serving.

Nutritional Information (per serving)
Calories 157.0, Total Fat 9.6 g, Saturated Fat 2.8 g,
Total Carbs 9.5 g, Dietary Fiber 3.4 g, Sugars 4.3 g, Protein 10.5 g

White Garlic Portabella Pizzas

Servings: 4
Prep Time: 10 minutes
Cook Time: 15 minutes

Ingredients
8 large portabella mushroom caps

2 tablespoons olive oil

5 cloves garlic

1 cup crème fraiche

½ cup Parmesan cheese

½ teaspoon salt

1 teaspoon coarse ground black pepper

1 cup artichoke hearts (canned or frozen), chopped

½ cup fresh basil, chopped

1 cup goat cheese

Directions
1. Begin by preheating the broiler.
2. Heat a large skillet over medium heat.
3. Brush the mushroom caps with olive oil on both sides and place them in the preheated skillet. Cook for approximately 3 minutes per side, or until tender but firm.
4. Remove the mushroom caps from the skillet and set them aside.
5. Add the remaining olive oil to the skillet, along with the garlic.
6. Cook the garlic, stirring frequently, for 2 minutes.

7. Add the crème fraiche, Parmesan cheese, salt, and coarse ground black pepper. Mix well and cook over medium heat for 2-3 minutes.
8. Spoon the white garlic sauce into the gill side of each of the mushroom caps.
9. Top each with the artichoke hearts, basil, and goat cheese.
10. Place the portabella pizzas under the broiler for 3-5 minutes, or until the tops are golden brown.
11. Serve immediately.

Nutritional Information (per serving)
Calories 395.5, Total Fat 31.9 g, Saturated Fat 16.9 g,
Total Carbs 13.4 g, Dietary Fiber 7.4 g, Sugars 4.3 g, Protein 17.4 g

Cajun Fish Taco Bowls

Servings: 4
Prep Time: 10 minutes
Cook Time: 10 minutes

Ingredients
1 tablespoon Cajun spice mix

1 tablespoon smoked paprika

½ teaspoon dry mustard powder

½ teaspoon salt

1 teaspoon coarse ground black pepper

1 pound tilapia fillets

1 tablespoon olive oil

2 cups cooked quinoa

1 cup red cabbage, shredded

½ cup pickled red onion (no sugar added)

1 cup fresh corn kernels

1 avocado, chopped

½ cup plain yogurt

¼ cup fresh cilantro, chopped

Directions
1. Mix together the Cajun spice mix, smoked paprika, mustard powder, salt, and black pepper.
2. Season both sides of each tilapia fillet liberally with the spice mixture.
3. Heat the olive oil in a skillet over medium heat.

4. Add the fish and cook for 3-4 minutes per side, or until cooked through. Remove the tilapia from the skillet and place it on a cutting board.
5. Cut the cooked fish into cubes.
6. Divide the cooked quinoa among serving bowls.
7. Top each bowl with red cabbage, pickled red onion, fresh corn kernels, and the Cajun fish.
8. Garnish with avocado, plain yogurt, and cilantro before serving.

Nutritional Information (per serving)
Calories 391.5, Total Fat 15.1 g, Saturated Fat 2.3 g,
Total Carbs 36.9 g, Dietary Fiber 8.4 g, Sugars 6.4 g, Protein 32.0 g

Pork in Mango Habanero Sauce

Servings: 4
Prep Time: 10 minutes
Cook Time: 15 minutes

Ingredients
1 pound pork tenderloin or roast, sliced into thin stirps

1 tablespoon coconut oil

1 cup red bell pepper, sliced

1 cup yellow bell pepper, sliced

1 cup Vidalia onion, sliced

2 cloves garlic, crushed and minced

2 cups unsweetened coconut milk

1 cup green salsa (no sugar added)

½ cup plain yogurt

1 habanero pepper, seeded and minced

1 cup mango, chopped

½ cup unsweetened shredded coconut

2 tablespoons lime juice

1 teaspoon ground cumin

¼ cup fresh basil, chopped

½ teaspoon salt

½ teaspoon black pepper

2 cups cooked brown rice for serving

Directions

1. Heat the coconut oil in a large skillet over medium heat.
2. Add the sliced pork and cook for 3-5 minutes, or until browned and mostly cooked through.
3. Using a slotted spoon, remove the pork from the skillet and set it aside.
4. Add the red bell pepper, yellow bell pepper, Vidalia onion, and garlic to the skillet. Cook, stirring frequently for approximately 5 minutes, or until the vegetables are tender.
5. Quickly combine the coconut milk, green salsa, plain yogurt, habanero pepper, mango, unsweetened shredded coconut, lime juice, cumin, basil, salt, and black pepper in a blender. Pulse until a sauce forms.
6. Place the cooked pork back into the skillet with the vegetables.
7. Add the blender sauce into the skillet and cook over medium heat until warmed through.
8. Serve immediately over brown rice.

Nutritional Information (per serving)

Calories 530.4, Total Fat 21.9 g, Saturated Fat 12.5 g,
Total Carbs 44.6 g, Dietary Fiber 5.7 g, Sugars 11.7 g, Protein 39.6 g

Santa Fe Turkey Burger Salad

Servings: 6
Prep Time: 15 minutes
Cook Time: 10 minutes

Ingredients

1 pound ground turkey

1 teaspoon salt

1 teaspoon black pepper

1 teaspoon onion powder

1 teaspoon ground cumin

1 cup pepper jack cheese, shredded

4 cups romaine lettuce, chopped

2 cups cherry tomatoes, halved

1 cup fresh corn kernels

1 avocado, cubed

½ cup low fat mayonnaise

½ cup plain yogurt

1 tablespoon sriracha

¼ cup red onion, finely diced

1 tablespoon rice vinegar

¼ cup fresh cilantro, chopped

Directions

1. Spray a large skillet with cooking spray.
2. Add the ground turkey and season it with the salt, black pepper, onion powder, and ground cumin. Cook over medium heat, stirring frequently, until it is browned and cooked through.
3. Use a slotted spoon to remove the cooked meat from the skillet, and set it aside to cool slightly.
4. Meanwhile, combine the pepper jack cheese, romaine lettuce, cherry tomatoes, fresh corn and avocado in a large bowl.
5. Add the ground turkey to the bowl and toss gently to mix.
6. In a separate bowl, whisk together the mayonnaise, plain yogurt, sriracha, red onion, rice vinegar, and fresh cilantro.
7. Pour the dressing over the salad and toss until the dressing is worked through.
8. Cover and refrigerate for at least 30 minutes before serving.

Nutritional Information (per serving)
Calories 432.6, Total Fat 32.9 g, Saturated Fat 4.6 g,
Total Carbs 12.4 g, Dietary Fiber 3.7 g, Sugars 2.4 g, Protein 24.2 g

Polynesian Chicken Nuggets

Servings: 4
Prep Time: 15 minutes plus refrigeration
Cook Time: 15 minutes

Ingredients
¼ cup fresh orange juice

½ cup fresh pineapple juice

¼ cup low sodium soy sauce

2 tablespoons kumquats, finely chopped

3 cloves garlic, crushed and minced

1 tablespoon crushed red pepper flakes

1 pound boneless, skinless chicken breast, cubed

½ cup coconut flour

1 egg, lightly beaten

1 cup unsweetened, shredded coconut

2 tablespoons coconut oil, melted

½ teaspoon salt

½ teaspoon black pepper

Directions
1. In a large bowl or food storage bag, combine the fresh orange juice, fresh pineapple juice, low sodium soy sauce, kumquats, garlic, and crushed red pepper flakes. Mix well.
2. Add the cubed chicken to the marinade and stir. Cover and refrigerate for 2 hours.
3. Preheat the oven to 400°F and line a baking sheet with aluminum foil.

29

4. Remove the chicken from the marinade, and set it aside on a plate lined with paper towel.
5. Place the remaining marinade in a small saucepan and set it aside.
6. Set up three bowls, one that contains the coconut flour, a second that contains the beaten egg, and a third that contains the unsweetened, shredded coconut.
7. Take each piece of chicken, dust it in the coconut flour then dip it into the egg before liberally coating it with the shredded coconut.
8. Place the nuggets on the baking sheet.
9. Once all the chicken has been coated, drizzle the melted coconut oil over the nuggets and toss gently.
10. Spread the nuggets out evenly on the baking sheet and place them in the oven.
11. Bake for 15-17 minutes, depending on the size of the pieces, until the chicken is cooked all the way through.
12. While the chicken nuggets are in the oven, place the reserved marinade in a saucepan on the stovetop over medium-high heat. Cook, stirring frequently, until the liquid comes to a boil for 1-2 minutes. Reduce the heat to medium low and cook for 5 minutes. Remove the pan from the heat and set it aside to allow the sauce to cool slightly.
13. Remove the chicken nuggets from the oven and season them with salt and black pepper.
14. Serve the nuggets with warm dipping sauce.

Nutritional Information (per serving)
Calories 384.1, Total Fat 22.9 g, Saturated Fat 16.8 g,
Total Carbs 17.4 g, Dietary Fiber 5.8 g, Sugars 7.8 g, Protein 29.7 g

No Noodle Lasagna Cups

Servings: 4
Prep Time: 15 minutes
Cook Time: 45 minutes

Ingredients
1 tablespoon olive oil

1 cup green bell pepper, chopped

1 cup red onion, chopped

4 cups fresh spinach, torn

8 ounces lean ground beef

3 cloves garlic, crushed and minced

½ teaspoon salt

1 teaspoon coarse ground black pepper

4 large, firm tomatoes

2 cups sugar free tomato sauce

1 tablespoon Italian seasoning

1 cup ricotta cheese

1 cup fresh mozzarella cheese, thinly sliced

½ cup Asiago cheese, shredded

¼ cup fresh basil, chopped

Directions
1. Heat the olive oil in a skillet over medium heat.
2. Add the green bell pepper and red onion. Sauté the mixture for approximately 5 minutes before adding in the spinach.
3. Continue cooking until the spinach begins to wilt.

4. Use a slotted spoon to remove the mixture from the skillet, and set it aside.
5. Add the ground beef and garlic to the skillet, and season with the salt and black pepper.
6. Cook, stirring frequently, until the meat is browned.
7. While the meat is browning, cut each of the tomatoes in half and scoop out the center flesh, leaving a little more than ¼ inch of shell. Reserve the insides.
8. Drain off any excess grease from the cooked meat.
9. Add the sautéed vegetable mixture back into the skillet with the meat, along with the insides of the tomatoes, and stir.
10. Next, add the tomato sauce and Italian seasoning. Heat over medium-low heat, stirring occasionally, until warmed through.
11. While the meat sauce is simmering, preheat the oven to 400°F and lightly oil a baking dish.
12. Spoon enough sauce into each tomato half to fill it about halfway.
13. Then add a spoonful of ricotta cheese, followed by more sauce, and finally a layer of fresh mozzarella cheese.
14. Place the tomato halves in the baking dish and place them in the oven.
15. Bake for 20-25 minutes, and then carefully remove the dish from the oven.
16. Sprinkle Asiago cheese and fresh basil over each tomato and place the dish back in the oven for 5 minutes.
17. Let sit for 5 minutes before serving.

Nutritional Information (per serving)
Calories 510.5, Total Fat 31.0 g, Saturated Fat 14.3 g,
Total Carbs 28.0 g, Dietary Fiber 5.6 g, Sugars 6.7 g, Protein 34.0 g

Quick Cajun Scallops over Wilted Greens

Servings: 4
Prep Time: 10 minutes
Cook Time: 20 minutes

Ingredients

1 teaspoon cayenne pepper sauce

2 teaspoons lemon juice

1 pound sea scallops

¼ cup coconut flour

1 tablespoon Cajun seasoning

½ teaspoon salt

1 tablespoon olive oil

4 ounces pancetta, cubed

¼ cup shallots, minced

¼ cup apple cider vinegar

6 cups fresh spinach

1 tablespoon crushed red pepper flakes

Directions

1. Combine the cayenne pepper sauce and lemon juice, and then drizzle the mixture over the scallops.
2. In a bowl, combine the coconut flour, Cajun seasoning, and salt. Mix well.
3. Add the scallops to the Cajun flour mixture and toss to coat.
4. Heat the olive oil in a large skillet over medium heat.
5. Add the scallops to the skillet and cook 2-3 minutes per side, or until cooked through.

6. Remove the scallops from the skillet and place them on a plate. Tent a piece of aluminum foil to keep them warm.
7. Meanwhile, add the pancetta and shallots to the skillet used for the scallops and cook, stirring frequently, until the pancetta is browned.
8. Next, add the apple cider vinegar, stir and reduce for 2 minutes.
9. Add the spinach to the skillet and cook, stirring frequently, until the spinach begins to soften and wilt.
10. Stir in the crushed red pepper flakes and cook for an additional 1-3 minutes, stirring occasionally.
11. Divide the spinach among serving plates and top each with an equal portion of the scallops.

Nutritional Information (per serving)
Calories 275.5, Total Fat 13.3 g, Saturated Fat 3.6 g,
Total Carbs 10.6 g, Dietary Fiber 4.0 g, Sugars 0.2 g, Protein 27.5 g

Strawberry Pecan Salad with Balsamic Pork Tenderloin

Servings: 4
Prep Time: 15 minutes
Cook Time: 15 minutes

Ingredients

1 pound pork tenderloin medallions

½ teaspoon salt

½ teaspoon black pepper

1 teaspoon ground sage

1 tablespoon olive oil

¼ cup balsamic vinegar, divided

6 cups fresh salad greens

½ cup blue cheese crumbles

¼ cup pecans, chopped

2 tablespoons walnut oil

1 teaspoon stone ground mustard

1 cup fresh strawberries, sliced

½ cup scallions, sliced

Directions

1. Season the pork tenderloin with the salt, black pepper, and ground sage.
2. Heat the olive oil in a large skillet over medium heat.
3. Once the oil is hot, arrange the pork in the skillet and cook for 2-3 minutes per side.

4. Add all but approximately 1 tablespoon of the balsamic vinegar to the skillet.
5. Increase the heat to medium high just long enough for the balsamic vinegar to come to a boil.
6. Reduce the heat to low and simmer, turning the pork occasionally in the balsamic reduction, until the vinegar forms a thick, caramelized syrup over the pork.
7. While the balsamic vinegar is reducing, combine the salad greens, blue cheese crumbles, and pecans in a bowl.
8. Whisk together the remaining balsamic vinegar, walnut oil, and stone ground mustard.
9. Add the dressing to the bowl with the greens and toss to coat.
10. Remove the pork medallions from the skillet and let them rest for 5 minutes. Slice into smaller pieces, if desired.
11. Divide the salad greens among serving plates.
12. Top each portion with sliced strawberries, balsamic pork, and scallions before serving.

Nutritional Information (per serving)
Calories 456.5, Total Fat 30.0 g, Saturated Fat 7.1 g,
Total Carbs 7.1 g, Dietary Fiber 2.6 g, Sugars 2.4 g, Protein 38.9 g

Blackberry Chicken Salad

Servings: 4
Prep Time: 15 minutes
Cook Time: None

Ingredients
1 pound boneless, skinless chicken breast, cooked and cubed

½ cup celery, diced

½ cup red onion, diced

½ cup water chestnuts, chopped

1 cup fresh blackberries, halved

¼ cup light mayonnaise

¼ cup plain yogurt

1 tablespoon apple cider vinegar

1 tablespoon fresh rosemary, chopped

1 teaspoon lemon zest

½ teaspoon salt

½ teaspoon black pepper

Directions
1. In a large bowl, combine the chicken, celery, red onion, water chestnuts, and blackberries.
2. In another bowl, mix together the light mayonnaise, plain yogurt, apple cider vinegar, rosemary, lemon zest, salt, and black pepper. Using a whisk, mix until completely blended.
3. Add the dressing to the chicken mixture and stir, working the dressing through the salad as much as possible.
4. Cover and refrigerate for 2 hours before serving.

Nutritional Information (per serving)
Calories 267.8, Total Fat 11.2 g, Saturated Fat 2.2 g,
Total Carbs 12.7 g, Dietary Fiber 3.0 g, Sugars 5.4 g, Protein 28.2 g

Dinner Recipes

Citrus Scented Asparagus Risotto

Servings: 6
Prep Time: 10 minutes
Cook Time: 30 minutes

Ingredients

1 pound fresh asparagus, woody ends of the stems removed

4 cups vegetable broth

¼ cup butter

1 cup leek, thinly sliced

1 cup Arborio rice

½ cup dry white wine (optional)

2 tablespoons lemon zest

1 tablespoon lemon juice

1 cup freshly grated Asiago cheese

1 teaspoon sea salt

1 teaspoon coarse ground black pepper

½ cup scallions, sliced

Directions

1. Begin by bringing a large pot of lightly salted water to a boil. Submerge the asparagus and cook for approximately 3 minutes.
2. Remove the asparagus from the water and immediately submerge it in an ice bath for 2 minutes. Remove the asparagus from the ice bath and set it aside on a towel to dry.
3. Cut the asparagus into bite-sized pieces.
4. Place the vegetable broth in a large saucepan over medium heat. Heat the broth until it is steaming, then reduce the heat to low and keep it warm.
5. Place the butter in a large skillet over medium heat.
6. Add the leeks and sauté for 2-3 minutes.
7. Next, add the Arborio rice and cook, stirring frequently, until the rice is lightly browned and toasted.
8. Add the dry white wine (if using) to the skillet and cook for 1-2 minutes to let the wine reduce.
9. Take approximately ½ to 1 cup of the vegetable broth and add it to the skillet. Cook, stirring constantly, until the stock is absorbed. Continue adding the vegetable broth in this manner, waiting until each addition is completely absorbed before adding more.
10. After the second addition of vegetable broth, add the lemon zest and lemon juice.
11. When you have about 1 cup of broth left, add the asparagus.
12. When the risotto is close to being done, it will become tender with just a bit of chewiness and will take on a creamy texture. At this point, stir in the Asiago cheese, sea salt, and black pepper.
13. Serve immediately, garnished with fresh scallions.

Nutritional Information (per serving)

Calories 281.0, Total Fat 13.9 g, Saturated Fat 8.9 g,
Total Carbs 32.5 g, Dietary Fiber 2.0 g, Sugars 2.0 g, Protein 9.4 g

Goat Cheese and Walnut Stuffed Chicken Breasts

Servings: 4
Prep Time: 10 minutes
Cook Time: 20 minutes

Ingredients

1 pound boneless, skinless chicken breasts

½ teaspoon salt

1 teaspoon coarse ground black pepper

½ cup goat cheese

¼ cup pomegranate seeds

¼ cup walnuts, chopped

1 tablespoon fresh tarragon, chopped

1 tablespoon olive oil

1 tablespoon shallots, minced

2 tablespoons apple cider vinegar

2 tablespoons chicken broth

Directions

1. Begin by pounding the chicken breasts until each piece is approximately half an inch thick, then season each piece with salt and black pepper. Set them aside.
2. In a bowl, combine the goat cheese, pomegranate seeds, walnuts, and tarragon. Mix well.
3. Make a slit into the center of each chicken breast that goes down most of the length of each piece, and about three quarters of the way through to the other side.

4. Take the goat cheese mixture and spoon an equal amount into each cut in the chicken breasts. Spread the mixture into the chicken evenly. Secure the opening with wooden toothpicks.
5. Heat the olive oil in a skillet over medium heat.
6. Once the oil is hot, add the chicken breasts and cook for 6-7 minutes per side, or until cooked all the way through.
7. Remove the chicken from the skillet and keep it warm.
8. Meanwhile, add the shallots to the skillet and sauté for 2-3 minutes, or until tender.
9. Add the apple cider vinegar and chicken broth to the skillet and cook, stirring frequently, until the sauce deglazes and thickens.
10. Serve the chicken immediately, drizzled with the pan sauce.

Nutritional Information (per serving)
Calories 286.7, Total Fat 17.1 g, Saturated Fat 5.5 g,
Total Carbs 3.6 g, Dietary Fiber 0.9 g, Sugars 1.9 g, Protein 30.3 g

Horseradish Sandwich Steak with Tomatoes and White Beans

Servings: 4
Prep Time: 10 minutes
Cook Time: 15 minutes

Ingredients
½ cup low fat sour cream

2 tablespoons prepared horseradish

1 tablespoon fresh chives, chopped

1 pound thinly sliced sandwich steak

½ teaspoon salt

1 teaspoon coarse ground black pepper

½ teaspoon onion powder

1 tablespoon olive oil

2 cups cherry tomatoes, halved

2 cups fresh spinach, chopped

2 cloves garlic, crushed and minced

1 tablespoon fresh oregano, chopped

1 tablespoon fresh parsley, chopped

1 (15 ounce) can cannellini beans, rinsed and drained

Directions
1. In a bowl, whisk together the low fat sour cream, prepared horseradish, and chives. Mix well and set it aside.
2. Season the sandwich steak with salt, black pepper, and onion powder. Set it aside.
3. Place the olive oil in a large skillet over medium heat.

4. Add the tomatoes to the skillet and cook, stirring frequently, until the skin on the tomatoes begin to blister.
5. Next, add the spinach, garlic, oregano, and parsley. Cook for approximately 5 minutes, or until the spinach is wilted and the tomatoes are softened.
6. Add the cannellini beans to the skillet and cook, stirring frequently, until they are warmed through.
7. Transfer the bean and vegetable mixture to serving plates.
8. If necessary, spray the skillet with a little bit of cooking spray.
9. Add the seasoned sandwich steak to the skillet over medium heat and cook approximately 3-5 minutes, or until cooked through.
10. Remove the sandwich steak from the skillet and place it on top of the tomato and bean mixture.
11. Top with the creamy horseradish sauce before serving.

Nutritional Information (per serving)
Calories 352.2, Total Fat 12.1 g, Saturated Fat 4.4 g,
Total Carbs 26.4 g, Dietary Fiber 5.8 g, Sugars 0.7 g, Protein 34.8 g

Creamy Sweet Onion and Mushroom Chicken

Servings: 4
Prep Time: 10 minutes
Cook Time: 20 minutes

Ingredients
1 pound boneless, skinless chicken breast, sliced

½ teaspoon salt

1 teaspoon coarse ground black pepper

1 teaspoon Chinese five spice powder

1 tablespoon coconut oil

1 cup Vidalia onion, sliced

2 cups assorted mushrooms, sliced

½ teaspoon nutmeg

1 tablespoon Worcestershire sauce

1 tablespoon coconut flour

1 cup vegetable broth

½ cup crème fraiche

¼ cup fresh parsley, chopped

Directions
1. Season the chicken with salt, black pepper, and Chinese five spice powder.
2. Place the coconut oil in a large skillet over medium heat.
3. Place the chicken in the skillet and cook, stirring frequently, until cooked through.
4. Remove the chicken from the skillet to a platter. Tent with aluminum foil to keep the chicken warm.

5. Add the Vidalia onions to the skillet and cook for 5 minutes.
6. Next, add the mushrooms, nutmeg, and Worcestershire sauce, and cook for an additional 3 minutes, or until the mushrooms begin to soften.
7. Sprinkle the coconut flour over the vegetables and stir.
8. Add the vegetable broth to the skillet and increase the heat to medium high.
9. Once the liquid comes to a boil, reduce the heat to medium low and cook, stirring occasionally, until the sauce thickens.
10. Remove the skillet from the heat and stir in the crème fraiche.
11. Add the chicken back into the skillet and stir.
12. Serve garnished with fresh parsley.

Nutritional Information (per serving)
Calories 319.7, Total Fat 19.1 g, Saturated Fat 11.7 g,
Total Carbs 8.3 g, Dietary Fiber 2.6 g, Sugars 1.9 g, Protein 28.3 g

Garden Vegetables with Dijon Sauce over Quinoa

Servings: 4
Prep Time: 10 minutes
Cook Time: 20 minutes

Ingredients

1 pound asparagus, woody ends removed

1 cup dry quinoa

1 tablespoon olive oil, divided

1 cup red onion, sliced

3 cups zucchini, sliced

2 cups yellow squash, sliced

2 cups green beans, trimmed

1 teaspoon sea salt

1 teaspoon coarse ground black pepper

¼ cup shallots, minced

2 tablespoons apple cider vinegar

½ cup vegetable broth

¼ cup Dijon mustard

1 cup heavy cream

1 tablespoon fresh thyme, chopped

1 teaspoon lemon zest

Directions
1. Bring a large pot of lightly salted water to a boil.
2. Place the asparagus in the boiling water and cook for 3 minutes, or until vibrant green in color.
3. Remove the asparagus from the boiling water and immediately submerge it in an ice bath for 1-2 minutes.
4. Remove the asparagus from the ice bath and transfer to a towel-lined plate. Pat it dry and set it aside.
5. Prepare the quinoa according to the package instructions.
6. Next, pour three-quarters of the olive oil in a large skillet over medium heat.
7. Add the red onion and cook for 3 minutes, stirring frequently, until it begins to soften.
8. Next, add the zucchini, yellow squash, green beans, salt, and black pepper. Cook, stirring frequently, until the vegetables become firm tender, approximately 7-10 minutes.
9. While the vegetables are cooking, drizzle the remaining olive oil in a saucepan over medium heat.
10. Add the shallots and cook for 2 minutes.
11. Next, add the apple cider vinegar and reduce for 1-2 minutes.
12. Pour the vegetable broth, along with the Dijon mustard, into the saucepan. Increase the heat to medium high and heat the liquid until it is steamy.
13. Add the heavy cream to the saucepan and reduce the heat to low. Simmer, stirring occasionally, for 5 minutes. Add the fresh thyme.
14. Chop the blanched asparagus and add it to the skillet with the vegetables.
15. Pour the Dijon sauce over the vegetables and stir. Cook over medium-low heat until warmed through.
16. Mix the lemon zest into the quinoa.
17. Distribute the quinoa among serving dishes and top with the Dijon vegetable mixture to serve.

Nutritional Information (per serving)
Calories 519.4, Total Fat 28.8 g, Saturated Fat 14.3 g,
Total Carbs 54.2 g, Dietary Fiber 10.6 g, Sugars 6.6 g, Protein 13.1 g

Salsa Verde Chicken with Mango Avocado Salsa

Servings: 4
Prep Time: 15 minutes
Cook Time: 30 minutes

Ingredients

1 pound boneless, skinless chicken breasts

1 cup queso fresco cheese, crumbled

1 teaspoon salt

1 teaspoon black pepper

1 tablespoon olive oil

2 cups jarred salsa verde

1 avocado, chopped

1 mango, chopped

1 cup red onion, chopped

1 jalapeño pepper, minced

¼ cup fresh cilantro, chopped

1 tablespoon lime juice

Directions

1. Preheat the oven to 375°F.
2. Make a deep slit along the side of each chicken breast and stuff the opening with the queso fresco cheese. Close the slit with wooden toothpicks, and season the chicken with salt and black pepper.
3. Place the olive oil in a skillet over medium heat.
4. Add the chicken to the skillet and brown it for 3-4 minutes per side.

5. Transfer the chicken to a small baking dish, and pour the salsa verde over it.
6. Place the chicken in the oven and bake for 20 minutes, or until it is cooked all the way through.
7. While the chicken is baking, combine the avocado, mango, red onion, jalapeño pepper, cilantro, and lime juice. Mix well and set aside.
8. Remove the chicken from the oven and let it rest for 5 minutes before serving.
9. Serve the chicken garnished with the mango avocado salsa.

Nutritional Information (per serving)
Calories 387.1, Total Fat 20.6 g, Saturated Fat 7.0 g,
Total Carbs 18.1 g, Dietary Fiber 4.8 g, Sugars 7.6 g, Protein 33.7 g

Coconut Curried Shrimp

Servings: 4
Prep Time: 10 minutes
Cook Time: 15 minutes

Ingredients
1 pound shrimp, cleaned and deveined

2 teaspoons lime juice

½ teaspoon salt

1 tablespoon coconut oil

1 cup green bell pepper, sliced

1 cup sweet yellow onion, sliced

1 tablespoon Thai chili pepper, minced (optional)

2 cloves garlic, crushed and minced

2 tablespoons curry powder

1 teaspoon coriander

1 tablespoon freshly grated ginger

2 cups coconut milk

1 teaspoon lime zest

3 cups hot cooked brown rice

¼ cup unsweetened, shredded coconut, toasted

Directions
1. Sprinkle the shrimp with lime juice and season it with salt.
2. Melt the coconut oil in a large, deep skillet.
3. Add the green bell pepper, sweet yellow onion, Thai chili pepper, garlic, curry powder, coriander, and ginger.

4. Cook, stirring frequently, for 5 minutes, or until the vegetables are firm tender and fragrant.
5. Add the coconut milk and lime zest to the skillet and increase the heat to medium high.
6. Once the coconut milk comes to a low boil, add the shrimp to the sauce and cook for 3 minutes.
7. Reduce the heat to medium low and continue cooking for 4-6 minutes, or until the shrimp is cooked through.
8. Serve over hot cooked brown rice, and garnish with toasted coconut.

Nutritional Information (per serving)
Calories 396.5, Total Fat 12.2 g, Saturated Fat 8.0 g,
Total Carbs 44.6 g, Dietary Fiber 5.8 g, Sugars 1.5 g, Protein 27.8 g

Slow Cooker Caribbean Roast

Servings: 8
Prep Time: 15 minutes
Cook Time: 8 hours

Ingredients

2 pounds chuck or cross rib beef roast

1 teaspoon sea salt

1 teaspoon coarse ground black pepper

1 tablespoon Dijon mustard

¼ cup fresh pineapple juice

1 tablespoon crushed red pepper flakes

4 cloves garlic, crushed and minced

1 cup sweet yellow onion, sliced

2 cups red bell pepper, sliced

1 cup fresh pineapple chunks

½ cup beef broth

Directions

1. Season the roast with the sea salt and black pepper.
2. In a bowl, whisk together the Dijon mustard, pineapple juice, and crushed red pepper flakes.
3. Use a pastry brush to brush the sauce over the entire surface of the roast.
4. Pat the minced garlic onto the surface of the roast.
5. Place the roast in the middle of a slow cooker.
6. Surround the beef roast with the sweet yellow onion, red bell pepper, and fresh pineapple chunks.
7. Pour the beef broth into the slow cooker.
8. Cover and cook on low for 8 hours.

9. Remove the cover from the slow cooker and let the roast rest for 10 minutes.
10. Using two forks, shred the roast and mix with the vegetables and pineapple before serving.

Nutritional Information (per serving)
Calories 369.8, Total Fat 22.2 g, Saturated Fat 1.6 g,
Total Carbs 7.5 g, Dietary Fiber 1.0 g, Sugars 4.2 g, Protein 32.8 g

Slow Cooker Ethiopian Style Stew

Servings: 6
Prep Time: 15 minutes
Cook Time: 6 hours

Ingredients
2 pounds bone-in chicken pieces, skin removed

½ teaspoon salt

1 teaspoon coarse ground black pepper

1 teaspoon smoked paprika

1 teaspoon cayenne powder

1 teaspoon ground ginger

1 cup red onion, chopped

1 cup green bell pepper, chopped

1 cup canned garbanzo beans, rinsed and drained

2 teaspoons coconut oil, melted

1 tablespoon coconut flour

½ cup chicken broth

Directions
1. Season the chicken with the salt, black pepper, smoked paprika, cayenne powder, and ground ginger.
2. Place the chicken in a slow cooker.
3. In a bowl, combine the red onion, green bell pepper, and garbanzo beans.
4. Drizzle the melted coconut oil over the vegetables and sprinkle on the coconut flour. Toss to mix.
5. Add the vegetables into the slow cooker with the chicken.
6. Pour the chicken broth into the slow cooker.

7. Cover and cook on high for 6 hours.
8. Remove the lid from the slow cooker and let the chicken rest for 10 minutes.
9. Carefully remove the chicken and pull the meat off the bones. Discard the bones.
10. Place the chicken back in the slow cooker with the sauce and other ingredients, and stir to combine before serving.

Nutritional Information (per serving)
Calories 227.8, Total Fat 6.3 g, Saturated Fat 2.9 g,
Total Carbs 14.6 g, Dietary Fiber 3.5 g, Sugars 0.8 g, Protein 27.9 g

Mint Orange Lamb Patties

Servings: 4
Prep Time: 15 minutes
Cook Time: 10 minutes

Ingredients

½ cup Vidalia onion, chopped

2 cloves garlic, crushed and minced

1 tablespoon orange zest

¼ cup fresh mint, chopped

1 pound ground lamb

2 tablespoons low sodium soy sauce

2 tablespoons fresh orange juice

½ teaspoon salt

1 teaspoon coarse ground black pepper

Directions

1. In a blender or food processor, combine the onion, garlic, orange zest, and mint. Pulse until finely chopped and well blended.
2. In a bowl, combine the ground lamb with the mixture from the blender, as well as the soy sauce and orange juice. Use your hands to mix well.
3. Form the lamb mixture into four evenly-sized patties.
4. Preheat an indoor or outdoor grill over medium heat.
5. Season the patties with salt and black pepper.
6. Place the patties on the preheated grill and cook for 4-5 minutes per side, depending upon thickness, until cooked through.
7. Remove the patties from the grill and let them rest for 5 minutes before serving.

Nutritional Information (per serving)

Calories 335.1, Total Fat 26.6 g, Saturated Fat 11.6 g,
Total Carbs 3.1 g, Dietary Fiber 0.4 g, Sugars 0.8 g, Protein 19.6 g

Pork and Cabbage Skillet Stir Fry

Servings: 4
Prep Time: 10 minutes
Cook Time: 15 minutes

Ingredients

1 pound ground pork

3 cloves garlic, crushed and minced

1 tablespoon freshly grated ginger

1 cup cremini mushrooms, sliced

2 cups napa cabbage, shredded

2 cups bok choy, shredded

¼ cup low sodium soy sauce

1 tablespoon sesame oil

1 teaspoon coarse ground black pepper

2 cups hot cooked rice

¼ cup scallions, sliced

Directions

1. Place the ground pork and garlic in a large skillet. Cook, stirring frequently, over medium heat for 5 minutes.
2. Add the ginger and mushrooms. Cook for an additional 3 minutes.
3. Next, add the napa cabbage and bok choy. Continue cooking while stirring.
4. Add the low sodium soy sauce, sesame oil, and black pepper. Cook for an additional 3-5 minutes, or until the pork is cooked through and the cabbage is tender.
5. Serve over hot cooked rice, garnished with sliced scallions.

Nutritional Information (per serving)

Calories 492.9, Total Fat 28.1 g, Saturated Fat 9.5 g,
Total Carbs 25.6 g, Dietary Fiber 2.0 g, Sugars 0.4 g, Protein 33.8 g

Vegetables and Side Dishes

Sesame Cashew Bok Choy

Servings: 4
Prep Time: 5 minutes
Cook Time: 10 minutes

Ingredients
1 tablespoon sesame oil

1 cup sweet onion, sliced

1 pound bok choy, chopped

1 tablespoon freshly grated ginger

1 tablespoon ponzu sauce

¼ cup cashews, chopped

½ teaspoon coarse ground black pepper

Directions
1. Heat the sesame oil in a large skillet over medium heat.
2. Add the onions and cook for 2 minutes.
3. Next, add the bok choy and ginger. Cook, stirring frequently, for an additional 2 minutes.
4. Add the ponzu sauce, cashews, and black pepper. Cook, stirring gently, until the bok choy is coated with sauce, tender, and slightly wilted.
5. Remove from the heat and serve immediately.

Nutritional Information (per serving)
Calories 107.1, Total Fat 7.4 g, Saturated Fat 1.3 g,
Total Carbs 8.5 g, Dietary Fiber 1.0 g, Sugars 0.8 g, Protein 3.9 g

Jalapeño Blue Slaw

Servings: 6
Prep Time: 15 minutes plus 2 hours refrigeration
Cook Time: None

Ingredients
2 cups red cabbage, shredded

2 cups green cabbage, shredded

1 cup carrot, shredded

1 cup onion, thinly sliced

1 jalapeño pepper, seeded and chopped (adjust to suit tastes)

¼ cup mayonnaise

½ cup plain low fat yogurt

2 tablespoons apple cider vinegar

¼ cup blue cheese crumbles

Directions
1. In a large bowl, combine the red cabbage, green cabbage, carrot, onion, and jalapeño. Toss to mix.
2. In a small bowl, combine the mayonnaise, plain yogurt, and apple cider vinegar. Whisk together until well blended.
3. Stir the blue cheese crumbles into the dressing.
4. Pour the dressing over the slaw mix and toss to coat.
5. Cover and refrigerate for 2 hours before serving.

Nutritional Information (per serving)
Calories 126.9, Total Fat 8.8 g, Saturated Fat 2.3 g,
Total Carbs 9.4 g, Dietary Fiber 2.3 g, Sugars 3.5 g, Protein 3.7 g

Grilled Asiago Zucchini

Servings: 4
Prep Time: 10 minutes
Cook Time: 5 minutes

Ingredients

1 pound zucchini

1 tablespoon olive oil

2 cloves garlic, crushed and minced

1 teaspoon lemon juice

1 teaspoon lemon zest

½ teaspoon salt

1 teaspoon coarse ground black pepper

¼ cup freshly grated Asiago cheese

Directions

1. Begin by preheating your broiler and an indoor or outdoor grill over medium heat.
2. Slice the ends off the zucchini, and then slice the zucchini lengthwise into approximately ¼-inch thick slices.
3. In a small bowl, whisk together the olive oil, garlic, lemon juice, and lemon zest.
4. Liberally brush the olive oil mixture over both sides of each piece of zucchini.
5. Season the zucchini with salt and black pepper.
6. Place the zucchini on the grill and cook for 2-3 minutes per side.
7. Remove the zucchini from the grill and place it on a foil-lined baking sheet.
8. Sprinkle the Asiago cheese over the zucchini and place it under the broiler for 1 minute.
9. Serve immediately.

Nutritional Information (per serving)

Calories 104.6, Total Fat 8.1 g, Saturated Fat 3.5 g,
Total Carbs 4.5 g, Dietary Fiber 1.6 g, Sugars 1.9 g, Protein 4.7 g

Eggplant Basil Rolls

Servings: 6
Prep Time: 10 minutes
Cook Time: 35 minutes

Ingredients
1 large eggplant

1 teaspoon salt, divided

1 tablespoon olive oil

½ cup goat cheese

½ cup provolone cheese, shredded

1 egg

½ cup fresh basil, chopped

2 cloves garlic, crushed and minced

1 cup sugar free tomato sauce

½ cup freshly grated Parmesan cheese

Directions
1. Preheat the oven to 350°F and lightly oil an 8x8 baking dish.
2. Slice the ends off the eggplant and then slice the eggplant lengthwise into ¼-inch thick pieces.
3. Lay the eggplant out on a towel and sprinkle it with half the salt. Flip the slices over and sprinkle the other side with the remaining salt. Let it sit for about 10 minutes to draw out the excess moisture.
4. Heat the olive oil in a large skillet over medium heat.
5. Brush the salt off the eggplant and place the eggplant in the skillet.

6. Cook for 1-2 minutes per side, or until lightly browned and softened.
7. Remove the eggplant from the skillet and set it aside.
8. In a bowl, combine the goat cheese, provolone cheese, egg, basil, and garlic.
9. Spread the mixture over each piece of eggplant and then roll each piece, starting on a short edge.
10. Place the eggplant rolls in the baking dish.
11. Cover the eggplant with the sugar free tomato sauce.
12. Place the baking dish in the oven and bake for 25 minutes.
13. Remove the baking dish from the oven, sprinkle the Parmesan cheese over the top and then bake for an additional 5 minutes.

Nutritional Information (per serving)
Calories 170.7, Total Fat 10.8 g, Saturated Fat 5.5 g,
Total Carbs 9.3 g, Dietary Fiber 2.9 g, Sugars 1.9 g, Protein 10.5 g

Skillet Creamed Spinach and Fennel

Servings: 4
Prep Time: 10 minutes
Cook Time: 10 minutes

Ingredients

1 tablespoon olive oil

1 cup fennel, thinly sliced

10 cups fresh spinach, torn

½ teaspoons salt

1 teaspoon black pepper

1 teaspoon nutmeg

½ cup goat cheese

½ cup crème fraiche

½ cup walnuts, chopped

Directions
1. Heat the olive oil in a skillet over medium heat.
2. Add the fennel and cook, stirring frequently, for 3-4 minutes, or until it becomes tender.
3. Add the spinach to the skillet and cook for 5 minutes, or until wilted. Season the mixture with salt, black pepper, and nutmeg, and stir.
4. Add the goat cheese and crème fraiche to the skillet and stir until creamy and melted.
5. Reduce the heat to low and let it simmer for 5 minutes.
6. Serve garnished with chopped walnuts.

Nutritional Information (per serving)
Calories 299.9, Total Fat 27.8 g, Saturated Fat 10.5 g,
Total Carbs 7.5 g, Dietary Fiber 3.3 g, Sugars 1.8 g, Protein 8.3 g

Warm and Spicy Brussels Sprouts

Servings: 6
Prep Time: 5 minutes
Cook Time: 10 minutes

Ingredients

2 tablespoons butter

6 cups Brussels sprouts, shredded

½ teaspoon sea salt

1 teaspoon coarse ground black pepper

1 teaspoon nutmeg

½ teaspoon cinnamon

¼ teaspoon cayenne powder

1 teaspoon orange zest

¼ cup orange juice

¼ cup pecans, chopped

Directions

1. Heat the butter in a large skillet over medium heat.
2. Add the Brussels sprouts and sauté for 3 minutes.
3. Add the sea salt, black pepper, nutmeg, cinnamon, cayenne powder, orange zest, and orange juice.
4. Continue cooking for an additional 5 minutes, or until the orange juice reduces and the sprouts become lightly browned and caramelized.
5. Remove the skillet from the heat and stir in the pecans before serving.

Nutritional Information (per serving)

Calories 110.7, Total Fat 7.7 g, Saturated Fat 2.8 g,
Total Carbs 9.6 g, Dietary Fiber 3.8 g, Sugars 3.0 g, Protein 3.5 g

Easy Italian Artichoke Salad

Servings: 6
Prep Time: 15 minutes plus refrigeration
Cook Time: None

Ingredients

2 cups canned artichoke hearts, drained and chopped

½ cup red onion, chopped

½ cup roasted red pepper, chopped

4 ounces capicola, chopped

2 cups cooked quinoa

¼ cup fresh basil, chopped

½ cup fresh parsley, chopped

1 cup tomatoes, chopped

¼ cup olive oil

¼ cup balsamic vinegar

Directions

1. In a bowl, combine the artichoke hearts, red onion, roasted red pepper, capicola, and quinoa. Mix well.
2. Add the basil, parsley, and tomatoes to the salad and gently fold them in.
3. Whisk together the olive oil and balsamic vinegar. Pour the dressing over the salad and toss gently to incorporate.
4. Cover and refrigerate for at least 30 minutes before serving.

Nutritional Information (per serving)

Calories 232.4, Total Fat 10.6 g, Saturated Fat 1.7 g,
Total Carbs 27.3 g, Dietary Fiber 4.4 g, Sugars 0.8 g, Protein 9.0 g

Creamy Portabella and Sundried Tomato Sauté

Servings: 4
Prep Time: 5 minutes
Cook Time: 10 minutes

Ingredients

8 ounces bacon, chopped

4 cups portabella mushrooms, sliced

3 cloves garlic, crushed and minced

½ cup sundried tomatoes, chopped

¼ cup heavy cream

½ cup Brie cheese, cubed

¼ cup freshly grated Parmesan cheese

Directions

1. Place the bacon in a large skillet over medium heat.
2. Cook the bacon, stirring frequently, until browned and lightly crispy. Drain any excess grease.
3. Add the portabella mushrooms, garlic, and sundried tomatoes to the skillet. Cook, stirring frequently, until the mushrooms soften, approximately 3-5 minutes.
4. Add the heavy cream and Brie to the skillet and cook, stirring constantly, until the cream is absorbed and the Brie is melted.
5. Add the Parmesan to the skillet and stir.
6. Serve immediately.

Nutritional Information (per serving)

Calories 217.8, Total Fat 16.6 g, Saturated Fat 9.3 g,
Total Carbs 6.8 g, Dietary Fiber 1.7 g, Sugars 3.9 g, Protein 12.8 g

Desserts

Tropical Banana Cookies

Servings: 18
Prep Time: 10 minutes plus refrigeration
Cook Time: 10 minutes

Ingredients

2 cups almond flour

1 cup rice flour

1 teaspoon baking soda

½ teaspoon salt

1 teaspoon coriander

1 teaspoon cinnamon

¼ cup coconut oil

1 vanilla bean

1 egg, beaten

1 egg white

½ cup banana, mashed

½ cup fresh pineapple chunks

1 cup unsweetened shredded coconut

¼ cup raisins, chopped

1 cup cashews, chopped

Directions

1. In a bowl, combine the almond flour, rice flour, baking soda, salt, coriander, and cinnamon.
2. In a separate bowl, combine the coconut oil, the scraped insides of the vanilla bean, the egg, egg white, and banana. Use an electric mixer on low to blend the ingredients together.
3. Working in two to three increments, add the dry ingredients into the wet ingredients.
4. Stir in the pineapple, unsweetened shredded coconut, raisins, and cashews.
5. Cover and refrigerate for at least 1 hour, or until the dough is firm.
6. Preheat the oven to 350°F and line a baking sheet with parchment paper or aluminum foil.
7. Drop spoonfuls of the cookie dough onto the baking sheet, leaving about 1-2 inches between each cookie.
8. Place the baking sheet in the oven and bake for 8-10 minutes, or until the cookies are golden brown.
9. Remove the cookies from the oven and let them cool before serving.

Nutritional Information (per serving)
Calories 214.7, Total Fat 15.4 g, Saturated Fat 5.9 g,
Total Carbs 16.9 g, Dietary Fiber 2.5 g, Sugars 3.7 g, Protein 5.3 g

Blood Orange Mojito Pops

Servings: 6
Prep Time: 10 minutes plus refrigeration
Cook Time: 7 minutes

Ingredients
1 ½ cups unsweetened coconut milk

1 tablespoon lime juice

¼ cup fresh mint, chopped

1 teaspoon pure vanilla extract

1 cup freshly squeezed blood orange juice

¼ cup blood orange wedges, chopped

Directions
1. In a bowl, combine the unsweetened coconut milk, lime juice, mint. and vanilla extract. Mix well and place in the refrigerator until ready to use.
2. Place the blood orange juice and the chopped wedges in a blender. Pulse for 20 seconds.
3. Pour the blood orange mixture into a small saucepan.
4. Over medium to medium-high heat, bring the liquid to a boil. Boil for 1-2 minutes, then reduce the heat to low and simmer for 5 minutes.
5. Remove the saucepan from the heat and allow the liquid to cool.
6. Once the liquid has cooled, add it to the coconut milk mixture and stir.
7. Pour the mixture into popsicle molds and place them in the freezer for at least 4 hours, or until firm.

Nutritional Information (per serving)
Calories 33.0, Total Fat 1.2 g, Saturated Fat 1.0 g,
Total Carbs 5.5 g, Dietary Fiber 0.5 g, Sugars 4.4 g, Protein 0.4 g

Georgia Peach Frozen Yogurt

Servings: 4
Prep Time: 10 minutes
Cook Time: None

Ingredients

4 cups peach slices, frozen

½ cup plain low fat yogurt

¼ cup orange juice

1 teaspoon freshly grated ginger

½ teaspoon cinnamon

Directions

1. In a blender, combine the frozen peaches, yogurt, orange juice, ginger, and cinnamon. Blend until creamy.
2. Transfer the mixture to a covered container and place it in the freezer for 15 minutes before serving.
3. Serve in chilled glasses.

Nutritional Information (per serving)

Calories 94.9, Total Fat 0.5 g, Saturated Fat 0.0 g,
Total Carbs 22.9 g, Dietary Fiber 3.9 g, Sugars 18.8 g, Protein 2.8 g

Yogurt Covered Coconut Cherries

Serves: 6
Prep Time: 10 minutes plus refrigeration
Cook Time: None

Ingredients
2 cups fresh cherries, halved and pitted

½ cup pineapple juice

1 cup sugar free vanilla Greek yogurt

½ teaspoon ground cinnamon

½ cup unsweetened, shredded coconut

Directions
1. Place the cherry halves and pineapple juice in a bowl. Cover and refrigerate for 1 hour.
2. Line a baking sheet or dish with parchment paper.
3. In a bowl, combine the yogurt and cinnamon.
4. Dip each cherry half into the yogurt and then place it on the baking sheet.
5. Once all the cherries have been dipped, liberally sprinkle the coconut over the cherries, patting it on if necessary to make it stick.
6. Place the baking sheet in the freezer and freeze for at least 2 hours before serving.

Nutritional Information (per serving)
Calories 80.7, Total Fat 4.5 g, Saturated Fat 4.0 g,
Total Carbs 9.5 g, Dietary Fiber 1.9 g, Sugars 7.3 g, Protein 1.6 g

Conclusion

There is no question that one of the most serious dietary issues we face today is the amount of processed flour and refined sugar the average diet contains. So many circumstances have led to our current, unhealthy diet habits. From the golden age when convenience foods were viewed as a novelty, to current times of hectic, overscheduled days – some of our taste buds have never learned what *real* food tastes like. Now is the time to make the change, to eliminate the bad stuff from your diet. Now is the time to finally know what it feels like to be healthy, to have energy and to enjoy wholesome and nutritious foods. It only takes two steps: eliminate the sugar, and eliminate the flour.

Honestly, once you work your way through this book and then use your own creativity to craft delicious sugar- and flour-free meals, you won't feel like you are missing a thing. In fact, you'll begin to feel like you've added something to your life instead. And you will have. You'll have added flavor, variety, vitality, and the chance for your body to finally repair itself and become its healthiest version yet.

Start today, start now. Go into your kitchen and clear out the junk – and then replace it with foods that will fuel and heal your body. Next, sit down with this book and plan out the meals of your healthy future, knowing that you will enjoy and feel completed satisfied with each and every one.

About the Author

Madison Miller is a nutritionist who is passionate about healthy eating and living a balanced lifestyle. She graduated in the late 1990s with a bachelor's degree in nutritional sciences. Madison has been working ever since as a nutritionist, consulting and helping people create a healthier lifestyle for themselves. She now shares her knowledge of nutrition, dieting, and healthy cooking through her books.

She loves exercising and doing research on nutrition to make healthy eating more exciting and diverse. Her books feature information about a lot of the diets there is around and easy ways to incorporate them into your life. She is also an avid cook, promoting recipes with fresh, wholesome ingredient that nourishes the body and the mind.

Madison lives in New York State with her husband and two young children.

More Books by Madison Miller

Here are some of Madison Miller's other cookbooks.

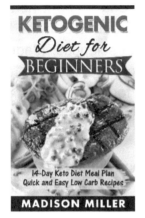
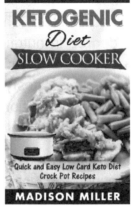
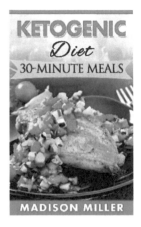

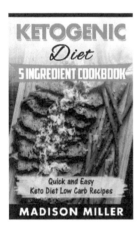
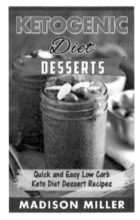
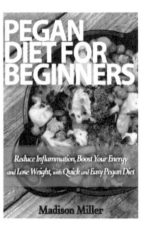

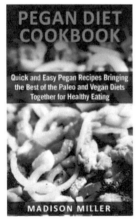
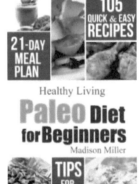
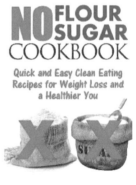

Appendix - Cooking Conversion Charts

1. Measuring Equivalent Chart

Type	Imperial	Imperial	Metric
Weight	1 dry ounce		28g
	1 pound	16 dry ounces	0.45 kg
Volume	1 teaspoon		5 ml
	1 dessert spoon	2 teaspoons	10 ml
	1 tablespoon	3 teaspoons	15 ml
	1 Australian tablespoon	4 teaspoons	20 ml
	1 fluid ounce	2 tablespoons	30 ml
	1 cup	16 tablespoons	240 ml
	1 cup	8 fluid ounces	240 ml
	1 pint	2 cups	470 ml
	1 quart	2 pints	0.95 l
	1 gallon	4 quarts	3.8 l
Length	1 inch		2.54 cm

*   Numbers are rounded to the closest equivalent

2. Oven Temperature Equivalent Chart

T(°F)	T(°C)
220	100
225	110
250	120
275	140
300	150
325	160
350	180
375	190
400	200
425	220
450	230
475	250
500	260

* $T(°C) = [T(°F)-32] * 5/9$

** $T(°F) = T(°C) * 9/5 + 32$

*** Numbers are rounded to the closest equivalent

Made in United States
Troutdale, OR
12/13/2023

15814239R00050